ESSENTIAL GUIDE TO WARTS

Understanding, Treating, and Preventing Warts: A Comprehensive Guide for Health and Wellness

DR. CASEY LOREN

DISCLAIMER

This book's content is only meant to be used for general informative purposes. Although the author has taken great care to ensure the content is accurate and thorough, no warranties or assurances on the information's accuracy, correctness, or reliability are provided. It is recommended that readers employ their own judgment and discretion when applying any material found in this book to their particular situation.

The information in this book is not intended to replace professional advice, nor is the author an expert in any of the subjects covered. It is recommended that readers consult with experienced professionals regarding any particular issues or concerns.

Any name that may be mentioned or referred in this book does not imply endorsement, recommendation, or relationship on the part of the author with any person, entity, good, website, or association. These references are made only for informational purposes and are not meant to be taken as recommendations or endorsements.

The information contained in this book may cause readers to suffer loss or damage, for which the author disclaims all obligation and accountability. The only people accountable for the decisions and actions taken by readers using the information presented are themselves.

Any names, characters, companies, locations, activities, occasions, and incidents referenced in this book are either made up or the result of the author's imagination. Any likeness to real people, living or dead, or to real things is entirely coincidental.

This book's content may change at any time, without prior notice, according to the author. The onus is on the reader to verify whether there have been any updates or revisions.

The reader accepts the conditions of this disclaimer by reading this book. Please do not read this book or use its contents if you do not agree to these terms.

Table of Contents

CHAPTER 1

GETTING TO KNOW WARTS

Warts, what are they?

Warts, which are produced by the human papillomavirus (HPV), are harmless skin growths. They can show up on any part of the body, including the hands, feet, face, or genitalia, and are easily identifiable by their rough texture. Touching an infected person's wart or touching a contaminated object, such as a razor or towel, might transmit the virus and cause a wart to grow on your skin.

Wart Types

Warts come in various forms and can cause discomfort depending on where they develop. Common warts tend to be on the hands and fingers, while plantar warts hurt when you walk and develop on your feet. Flat warts are small and smooth, and they often appear in clusters on your face, neck, or hands. Finally, there are genital warts, which are transmitted sexually and can show up anywhere from your genitalia to your surrounding areas.

What triggers warts

Warts are caused by the human papillomavirus (HPV), which infects the outer skin layer and triggers its fast growth, ultimately leading to the development of a wart. Various forms of warts can be caused by different strains of HPV. Factors that increase the risk of developing warts include having a compromised immune system, having cuts or scratches on the skin, and being in close contact with someone who has warts.

Who could be hurt?**

Warts can appear on anyone, but those who are more likely to get them include young people, those with compromised immune systems, nail biters, skin pickers, and those who have been near a wart carrier.

Typical misunderstandings regarding warts

Touching amphibians, such as frogs or toads, can produce warts, contrary to popular belief. The human papillomavirus (HPV) is responsible for the development and transmission of warts. The idea that over-the-counter medicines like duct tape or apple cider vinegar may magically eradicate warts is another common misunderstanding. These approaches have a chance of success for certain individuals, but they aren't foolproof and can occasionally lead to skin irritation or illness.

Diagnosing Warts

The look and location of warts on the body are the main criteria for diagnosing them. During a physical exam, a doctor may decide to biopsy a little piece of wart tissue to learn more about the condition. Dermoscopy is a tool that dermatologists may use to investigate warts further.

Difficulties linked to warts

Warts aren't dangerous in and of themselves, but they can annoy or hurt if they appear on places like the feet that carry a lot of weight. Complications like cellulitis or abscess formation can occur in extremely rare instances when warts get infected. Furthermore, some strains of HPV that cause genital warts can raise a woman's risk of cervical and other cancers.

The effect of warts on the emotions

Warts, especially those in sensitive regions or those that are quite noticeable, can cause a lot of distress for people. They have the potential to lower the quality of life by inducing feelings of shame, insecurity, and social anxiety. Warts can be emotionally taxing, but getting aid from healthcare providers or support groups can ease the burden.

Wart spread prevention

You can stop the spread of warts by being careful with your hygiene, not touching or picking at your warts, and not sharing things like razors or towels. Another way to lessen the likelihood of spreading genital warts is to use a condom whenever you engage in sexual activity. Vaccination against specific types of HPV also reduces the likelihood of genital warts and their consequences.

A look back at wart remedies

Warts have been surgically removed, frozen (cryotherapy), laser treated, and treated topically at various points in history.

Common ancient cures included scraping the wart with a coin or using plant extracts. Patients afflicted by warts have had better results as a result of more targeted and effective therapies made possible by scientific and technological advancements in the medical field.

CHAPTER 2

VARIOUS WART FORMS

Verruca vulgaris, or common warts

Human papillomavirus (HPV) causes common warts, which are non-cancerous skin growths also called verruca vulgaris. They show up on the fingers, hands, or nail beds and are usually little, rough, and elevated. Common warts can have a rough texture and a variety of colors, from flesh to grayish-brown. While innocuous in most cases, they may cause discomfort or embarrassment to certain people.

You can treat common warts with over-the-counter drugs that contain salicylic acid, freeze the wart off with cryotherapy, or even have it surgically removed if it's really bad. Keep in mind that although treatments can get rid of warts, they might not get rid of the HPV virus entirely, so warts can come back occasionally.

Plantar warts

The bottoms of the feet can get infected with plantar warts. They can be flat or slightly elevated, have a rough appearance, and sometimes contain black dots—which are blocked blood vessels—inside them. Since plantar warts can irritate the delicate nerves in the foot, they are most noticeable when one is walking or standing.

A few options for treating plantar warts include salicylic acid over-the-counter remedies, cryotherapy, laser therapy, or even small surgery. One way to stop the spread of plantar warts is to keep your feet clean and not go barefoot in public.

Flat warts, often known as verruca plana,

Clusters of tiny, smooth warts with flat tops are known as flat warts or verruca plana. The palms, knees, neck, and face are the most typical places to find them. Warts that are flat and not elevated at all tend to be flesh-colored or somewhat pink.

Flat warts can be treated with a variety of methods, including prescription drugs, cryotherapy, laser therapy, or topical medications containing salicylic acid or other keratolytic agents. Although adults are not immune to flat warts, they tend to manifest more frequently in younger people.

Varus deformities

Long, narrow warts called filiform warts typically show up on the face, neck, or in the areas surrounding the mouth and nose. In appearance, they resemble threads or fingers, and their color can range from flesh to brown or yellow. Although HPV-induced filiform warts are mostly harmless, their unsightly look can be a nuisance.

Cryotherapy, topical medicine, laser treatment, or even a little surgery can remove filiform warts. For accurate diagnosis and treatment of filiform warts, it is crucial to seek the advice of a healthcare practitioner.

Warts inside the mouth

Warts that grow all the way around or under the fingernails are called periungual warts. On top of being painful, they have the potential to alter the nail's texture and shape. People who bite their nails or have damaged cuticles are more likely to get periungual warts, which are caused by HPV.

Medication applied topically, cryotherapy, laser treatment, or surgical excision are all potential options for treating periungual warts. To stop periungual warts from getting worse or spreading, it's important to get them treated as soon as possible.

Condyloma acuminatum, often known as genital warts,

The growth of warts in the anal and genital regions is referred to as condyloma acuminatum or genital warts. Certain strains of HPV, which are transferred through sexual contact, are the source of these infections. Genital warts are unpleasant and irritating little pimples that might be flesh-colored or clusters of bumps.

Minor surgical treatments, cryotherapy, laser therapy, or topical medicine may be used to treat genital warts. Because genital warts can be a sign of an HPV infection, getting medical help for them is crucial. You may need to be monitored or given extra treatment.

Verruca vulgaris, or oral warts

Warts that appear on or near the mouth, lips, or throat are called oral warts or verruca vulgaris. They might take the form of clusters of bumps or little-raised lumps and are caused by HPV. When oral warts get in the way of eating or talking, they can be rather bothersome.

Surgical excision, cryotherapy, laser therapy, or topical medicine may be used to treat oral warts. Because oral warts can be a sign of a herpes simplex virus infection, it is crucial to see a doctor for a correct diagnosis and treatment.

Warts and seborrhoeic keratosis

Many people confuse seborrhoeic keratosis, a common non-cancerous skin growth, for warts. Although human papillomavirus (HPV) is the causative agent of warts, seborrhoeic keratosis is virus-free. Raised, waxy, brownish-black, or stuck-on seeming growths are the usual symptoms of seborrhoeic keratosis. They often do not cause any harm and are more prevalent in the elderly.

For cosmetic purposes or if they become irritating or unpleasant, surgical removal, cryotherapy, or laser therapy are all options for treating seborrhoeic keratoses.

Warts vs Molluscum contagiosum

As a result of infection with the molluscum contagiosum virus (MCV), molluscum contagiosum appears on the skin. The skin may develop tiny, dome-shaped lumps that resemble warts and are flesh-colored. But a different virus causes molluscum contagiosum, and that one usually spreads from person to person by skin-to-skin contact.

Molluscum contagiosum treatment options range from topical medicine to cryotherapy to small incisions in the skin. To diagnose and treat molluscum contagiosum correctly, it is necessary to distinguish it from warts.

Identifying uncommon varieties of warts

Although they may not be common, it is crucial to be aware of the following uncommon wart types:

1. Warts that grow on the tips of the fingers or the big toes are called digital warts.

2. **Ear warts:** Those that grow on the inside of the ear.

3. The growth of warts under or around the nails is known as subungual or periungual warts.

4. Warts that grow on the larynx (voice box) are called laryngeal warts.

5. **Plantar verrucous carcinoma:** This extremely rare and dangerous skin cancer might seem similar to plantar warts but needs expert medical care to be diagnosed and treated.

The key to effective treatment and management of uncommon wart types is early detection and accurate diagnosis. For uncommon or odd warts, it's best to consult a healthcare provider for advice.

CHAPTER 3
POSSIBLE ROOTS AND DANGERS

Warts and the Human Papillomavirus

The majority of cases of warts are caused by different types of the HPV virus. One common virus that can infect the outer layer of skin and cause it to grow quickly and develop into a wart is HPV. Some of the more than a hundred distinct kinds of human papillomavirus are more prone to causing warts than others. The following kinds of human papillomavirus (HPV) are the most prevalent ones: 1, 2, 3, 4, 27, and 29.

The Causes and Methods of HPV Transmission

High-risk papillomavirus (HPV) transmission occurs most often through close personal contact with an infected individual. Although this can happen when you're having sex, it's important to remember that not all types of HPV that cause warts can be transferred in this way. Sharing intimate objects like razors, towels, or other items with someone who has HPV can potentially spread the virus indirectly.

Hereditary Propensity for Warts

Warts may run in families and be inherited by certain people. As a result, they may be more prone to acquiring warts when exposed to HPV because their immune system isn't as strong.

Factors in the Environment That Can Cause Warts

Warts are more likely to appear in people who are exposed to specific environmental conditions. Some of these factors include being a frequent visitor to public areas prone to HPV transmission, such as swimming pools, locker rooms, shared showers, or residing in humid climates.

Warts and the Immune System:

Protecting oneself from HPV infections and warts relies heavily on a robust immune system. Warts can form more easily and stay longer or be more severe in people with compromised immune systems, such as those with HIV/AIDS, those receiving organ transplants and using immunosuppressive drugs, or those going through chemotherapy.

The Role of Gender and Age in Risk

Though they can develop at any age, warts disproportionately affect youth. This is because HPV infections tend to be more common in younger people as their immune systems are still developing. Nevertheless, warts are able to infect individuals of any age. Gender differences in anatomy and sexual behavior explain why some wart kinds, such as genital warts, affect one sex more frequently than the other.

Warts and Their Impact on the Workplace

Exposure to HPV and the resultant development of warts may be more common in certain employment. An increased risk of HPV infection may be present, for instance, in the healthcare industry, among childcare carers, and in vocations involving frequent skin-to-skin contact or handling contaminated equipment.

What You Can Do To Prevent Warts

The probability of having warts might be affected by specific lifestyle factors. Things like not washing hands often or discussing personal things are examples of bad hygiene practices. In addition, picking at warts or biting nails are two behaviors that can lead to the spread of the virus and the development of new warts.

Preventing Warts through Proper Hygiene

One way to lessen the likelihood of getting HPV and warts is to maintain adequate personal cleanliness. Some examples of this behavior include not sharing towels or razors and always washing one's hands after using the lavatory or swimming pool. Avoiding contact with warts and properly caring for wounds are other ways to prevent the transmission of HPV.

Common Misconceptions Regarding Wart Origins

It is not true that touching frogs or toads can produce warts; this is only one of many misconceptions about the causes of warts. Unlike toads and frogs, warts are caused by the human papillomavirus (HPV). The idea that warts can spread through hand-to-hand contact, like shaking hands, is likewise unfounded. Usually, to transmit HPV from one person to another, you need to come into direct touch with an infected area.

Warts can be better managed and treated, and the likelihood of infection can be lower, if people are aware of the many causes and risk factors linked with warts.

CHAPTER 4

MEDICAL EVALUATION AND DIAGNOSIS

Evaluation of Warts in the Clinic

To determine the presence, type, size, and location of warts, a comprehensive examination of the skin is conducted during a clinical examination. Dermatologists usually check the wart's texture and consistency by looking at it and, occasionally, touching it. They might also ask if you're experiencing any discomfort or itching because of the warts.

Warts Examined Through a Dermatologic Lens

Dermatoscopy allows for the non-invasive examination of skin lesions, such as warts. The procedure requires the use of a dermatoscope, a device that magnifies and lights the skin. This allows physicians to examine the wart's structures and patterns. By analyzing dermatoscopic characteristics such as vascular patterns and surface textures, this examination aids in differentiating warts from other skin disorders.

Possible Wart Diagnoses

Warts need to be differentiated from other skin disorders that could look similar to make a differential diagnosis. The benign and malignant lesions that fall under this category include skin tags, seborrhoeic keratosis, and molluscum contagiosum. To make a correct differential diagnosis, it is helpful to consider the patient's symptoms, history, physical features, and geographic location.

Recognising Warts at High Risk

Any wart that could cause problems or be an indication of a more serious health problem is considered a high-risk wart. Some examples of these are warts that develop quickly or come back, those that affect sensitive areas like the face or mucous membranes, and warts in people with impaired immune systems. To properly treat and follow up on warts, it is essential to identify those that pose a high risk.

Wart Treatment: When to Visit a Doctor

Warts should be treated by a doctor if they are painful, bleeding, itchy, or causing cosmetic issues. Also, a professional evaluation is necessary for people with high-risk warts or who are uncertain about self-treatment. It's crucial to consult a doctor if warts persist despite using over-the-counter remedies or if they reappear regularly.

Procedures and Tests for Wart Diagnosis

When diagnosing warts, it may be necessary to do a visual examination, dermatoscopy, biopsy (which is not often necessary for common warts), and viral testing (to confirm HPV infection in genital warts, for example). In addition to chemical therapies, dermatologists may diagnose and treat warts using cryotherapy (freezing), laser therapy, or other similar methods.

Visiting a Skin Specialist

For an accurate diagnosis, it is best to see a dermatologist. This is particularly true if the warts are persistent, spread, or otherwise difficult to treat. Specialized treatment, procedures like cryotherapy or laser therapy, and advice on self-care and prevention techniques are all things that dermatologists may offer.

Evaluation of Wart Patients' Mental Health

If a patient's quality of life or emotional well-being is significantly impacted by warts, a psychological evaluation may be in order. Healthcare providers can better assist their patients and send them to mental health specialists if necessary by using this assessment to detect wart-related anxiety, sadness, or body image disorders.

Patient Background and the Development of Warts

Understanding wart progression requires patient history, which includes past treatments, length of warts, and any related symptoms. Warts can be better monitored and treated by keeping track of their size, number, and appearance as they change over time.

Diagnosing Warts in Specific Groups

Variations in immune response and skin characteristics make wart diagnosis in special populations, such as immunocompromised patients, youngsters, and the elderly, very challenging. Different therapeutic considerations may be necessary for pediatric patients and the elderly, who may require a softer approach. Warts can be more severe or more widespread in immunocompromised people, who may need particular treatment.

This all-inclusive book goes over every single facet of wart evaluation, diagnosis, and treatment, stressing the significance of expert evaluation and tailored treatment according to patient traits and risk factors.

CHAPTER 4

WART TREATMENT ALTERNATIVES

Wart remedies available without a prescription

The initial line of defense against warts is frequently over-the-counter (OTC) medicines. The salicylic acid they often contain aids in the gradual disintegration of the wart tissue. The many formulations of these remedies include pads, liquids, ointments, and gels. For the best results, apply them consistently for a few weeks on your hands and feet if you have common warts.

Medication for warts that requires a prescription

If over-the-counter remedies fail or the warts are located in delicate locations, a dermatologist may recommend harsher medications. For example, a healthcare provider may recommend a topical medication like imiquimod to strengthen the immune system and combat the wart-causing virus, or cantharidin to induce blistering and have the wart surgically removed.

Wart eradication with cryotherapy (freezing)

The wart is treated with liquid nitrogen during cryotherapy, which causes it to blister and eventually fall off. It's usually done in a dermatologist's office and can take more than one session to get rid of it completely. Although cryotherapy effectively removes many kinds of warts, it is not without its risks, including potential discomfort, skin discoloration, and scarring.

Wart removal using electrosurgery and lasers

Warts can be surgically removed using electrosurgery or laser therapy, two medical procedures that employ light or heat radiation. They are usually done by medical experts and are reserved for larger or resistant warts. Anesthesia may be necessary for these procedures, and there are dangers such as infection or scarring, but they are precise and can reduce harm to adjacent skin.

A variety of topical and homeopathic therapies

Home therapies such as duct tape occlusion, apple cider vinegar, or tea tree oil are tried by some in addition to over-the-counter medications. Despite the amount of talk about these strategies, not everyone will find success with them. When dealing with widespread or chronic warts, it is crucial to seek the advice of a healthcare professional before trying any home cures.

Treatment of persistent warts with intralesional treatment

As part of intralesional therapy, a medicine is injected straight into the wart. Bleomycin and interferon are common agents used for this purpose because they trigger the immune system to attack the wart. Pain or inflammation at the injection site are possible side effects, but this focused method is great for obstinate warts that haven't responded to prior treatments.

Wart removal by surgical means

Surgical removal of big or persistent warts may be required. The wart will be surgically removed while the patient is under local anesthesia. Although it works, surgical excision leaves a scar and necessitates post-procedure wound care. Warts that are unsightly or haven't responded to other treatments are the usual candidates for this procedure.

Wart immunotherapy

Immunotherapy is a treatment for warts that works by stimulating the immune system to attack the virus that causes them. Several ways exist for this, such as injecting or applying chemicals like squaric acid dibutyl ester (SADBE) or candida antigen topically. Multiple rounds of immunotherapy may be necessary to achieve the best outcomes for treating resistant warts.

Anti-wart treatment regimens that include multiple modalities

A combination of treatments may be suggested for extremely extensive or persistent warts. Immunotherapy, cryotherapy, laser therapy, and other topical treatments could be used in combination. Better results for difficult warts may be possible with case-specific combination therapy.

Wart treatment counseling and support

It can be emotionally taxing to deal with warts, particularly if they come back or are persistent. Stress management, resolving issues related to one's looks or discomfort, and maintaining motivation throughout treatment can all benefit from counseling and assistance provided by healthcare providers. Those dealing with wart treatment may also find solace in joining a support group or an online forum where they may talk to others going through the same thing.

The overall strategy for treating warts is conditional upon variables such as the wart's kind, its location, and its reaction to the first treatments. The best way to manage warts is to see a doctor who can provide an accurate diagnosis and create a unique treatment plan for you.

CHAPTER 6

METHODS FOR PREVENTING WARTS

Practices in personal hygiene that can ward against warts

Avoiding the transmission of warts begins with practicing good hygiene. The following are some fundamental guidelines:

1. **Regular Handwashing:** It is extremely important to wash your hands frequently with soap and water, particularly after touching anything that could have touched warts.

2. **Refrain from Sharing Personal Items:** The virus that causes warts can be transmitted by sharing personal items such as towels, razors, and socks.

3. Warts are more likely to occur in wet conditions, therefore it's important to keep your skin dry and clean to lessen your chances of getting them.

4. You can stop the spread of warts by keeping them covered with a bandage if you have any.

Staying away from warts

You are more likely to get warts if you come into direct touch with them. I'll tell you what to do:

1. To reduce the likelihood of transmitting the virus, **Avoid Touching Warts**. This includes both your own and other people's warts.

2. **Protective Clothes:** To lessen the likelihood of coming into direct touch with surfaces that may be harboring the virus, it is advisable to wear protective footwear, such as flip-flops, when

visiting public spaces like swimming pools or gyms.

The Purpose of HPV Vaccination in Wart Prevention

The HPV vaccine is an important tool in the fight against warts:

1. Vaccination against human papillomavirus (HPV) lessens the probability of acquiring warts by protecting against specific strains of the virus.

2. **Healthcare Professional-Recommended Vaccination Schedule:** Vaccination against HPV should begin throughout adolescence or later if the doctor recommends it.

Enhancing the Immune System to Prevent Warts

Warts are less likely to occur in those with robust immune systems because the virus is more easily fought:

1. A healthy immune system is the result of a well-rounded diet that provides the body with the nutrients it needs.

2. Maintenance and proper functioning of the immune system depend on getting a sufficient amount of sleep.

3. If you want to keep your immune system strong, it's a good idea to exercise often.

4. Relaxation Methods: Regular use of relaxation techniques, such as yoga or meditation, can help keep the immune system in good working order.

Alterations to one's way of life that can ward off warts

Modifications to one's way of life can help reduce the likelihood of warts:

1. **Stop Smoking:** The immune system is weakened by smoking, which increases the risk of illnesses like warts.

2. **Controlling Alcohol Consumption:** Like other chemicals, too much alcohol can lower immunity, therefore it's best to drink in moderation.

Environmental measures to prevent warts

One way to lessen the likelihood of warts is to take environmental precautions:

1. A good way to limit the spread of the virus is to clean surfaces that come into touch with the skin regularly. This includes exercise equipment and shared showers.

2. You should not go barefoot in public places where the virus could be present, like public showers or locker rooms.

Sharing information about how to avoid warts

It is crucial to educate people on how to prevent warts:

1. **Sharing Information:** Spread the word about the significance of immunization, proper cleanliness, and avoiding coming into direct touch with warts.

2. Be a part of community health programs or campaigns that aim to educate people about how to prevent warts.

Ways to Travel While Minimising the Risk of Warts

To reduce the risk of contracting warts when traveling, take the following measures:

1. When you're going to areas with pools or shared showers, be sure to wear protective footwear, such as flip-flops or water shoes.

2. If you're staying in a shared room, it's extremely important that you not share towels or razors with other guests.

Avoiding the Recurrence of Warts

Constant attention is required to avoid wart recurrence:

1. **Skin Monitoring:** Keep an eye out for the appearance of new warts or changes to existing ones regularly.

2. Seek treatment immediately if you discover any new warts so they don't spread or return.

Prevention by monitoring and early identification

Important tactics for preventing warts include monitoring and early detection:

1. To find new warts or changes in old ones, it's a good idea to do self-exams of the skin regularly.

2. If you observe any irregularities, it is important to seek the advice of a healthcare expert so that you can be properly evaluated and treated.

Individuals can help improve public health by lowering their own risk of wart development and by spreading the word about these techniques to others.

CHAPTER 7

HANDLING INSTANCES OF RECURRENCE AND COMPLICACY

Untreated warts might lead to serious complications.

Many problems can arise from untreated warts, such as:

1. The human papillomavirus (HPV) is the causative agent of warts, and if left untreated, the virus can spread to other areas of the body or other persons through physical contact.

2. When warts expand in size or appear in painful places, like on the bottoms of feet or other weight-bearing areas, they can cause significant discomfort.

3. ***Cosmetic Considerations**: Warts, especially on more exposed regions like the hands

or face, can be embarrassing and make people feel self-conscious.

Wart-Related Secondary Infections

Secondary infections can develop when warts leave skin holes that bacteria and other organisms can easily exploit. Enhanced discomfort, redness, heat, swelling, and pus discharge are all indicators of an infection. To cure these infections, antibiotics need to be taken quickly.

Pain Control During Wart Removal

Oral pain medications, cold therapy (cryotherapy), and topical anesthetics are some of the pain management options that can be used while treating warts. Based on your pain tolerance, the size and location of the wart, and other factors, your healthcare practitioner can advise you on the best course of action.

Mental Health Assistance for People Living with Warts

Warts, particularly recurring or persistent ones, can be emotionally taxing to deal with. Patients who suffer from anxiety, humiliation, or frustration as a result of their illness can find relief through psychological support services like counseling or support groups.

Handling Wart Treatment Scarring

Scarring is rare after wart treatments, although it can happen, especially with more drastic methods like laser therapy or surgery. Minimizing the risk of scarring and promoting optimal healing can be achieved by proper wound care and regular follow-up with your healthcare professional.

Frequency of Occurrence and Risk Factors

Wart types, treatment efficacy, and personal variables including immune system health all contribute to the wart recurrence rate. Recurrence risk factors include unfinished therapy, neglecting underlying immune system disorders, and being exposed to HPV from infected people or untreated warts.

Methods for Stopping Warts from Coming Back

Complete adherence to treatment regimens, excellent personal hygiene, not sharing personal belongings (such as shoes or towels), and treatment of any underlying health issues that can lower the immune system are all crucial in reducing the likelihood of wart recurrences.

Dealing with Post-Wart Emotional Distress

Warts can damage a person's self-esteem and social interactions, which can cause emotional anguish that can persist even after therapy is effective. Overcoming these obstacles can be aided by maintaining psychological support and engaging in self-care techniques.

Treating Warts That Don't Go Away

It may be necessary to see a healthcare provider regularly for treatment and monitoring of persistent or chronic warts. These difficult cases can be better managed with combination therapy, treatments that stimulate the immune system, and frequent check-ups.

Complication Monitoring and Follow-Up Care

It is crucial to check for consequences like infections, scars, or recurrence during and after wart treatment with regular follow-up appointments. When necessary, your healthcare practitioner will set up follow-up visits and advise you on how to care for yourself after treatment.

Providers of holistic care for patients with warts can improve treatment outcomes, reduce the likelihood of complications, and boost patients' mental health by attending to all of these factors.

CHAPTER 8

VARIOUS NON-CONVENTIONAL MEDICAL PRACTICES

Natural Treatments for Warts

Warts are only one of several ailments that have traditionally been treated using herbal treatments. Garlic, aloe vera, and tea tree oil are three of the most common plants used to remove warts. The antiviral and immune-boosting qualities of these all-natural compounds make them promising candidates for the treatment of warts.

Wart Relieving Acupuncture and Acupressure

Traditional Chinese medicine practices like acupuncture and acupressure use the stimulation of certain places on the body to alleviate pain and speed up the healing process. Although there isn't a tonne of proof that these approaches remove warts, they do help some people deal with the pain and anxiety that comes with having warts.

Wart Treatment with Aromatherapy and Essential Oils

In aromatherapy, plant-based essential oils are used to enhance mental and physical health. Applying tea tree, lemon, or thuja oil physically or using it in aromatherapy sessions may help treat warts because of its antiviral characteristics.

A Guide to Homoeopathic Wart Treatments

To promote the body's inherent healing abilities, homeopathy employs extremely dilute chemicals. The homeopathic treatments Thuja occidentalis, Antimonium crudum, and Nitricum Acidum are commonly used to treat warts. The specific symptoms and constitution of the patient dictate which medications are prescribed.

Taking Nutrient Supplements to Treat Warts

Zinc, vitamin C, and echinacea are a few dietary supplements that may indirectly aid in the fight against warts by supporting immune function. Nevertheless, additional studies are required to confirm the efficacy of these supplements in managing warts.

Mind-Body Methods for Wart Management

If you suffer from anxiety or tension due to warts, mind-body treatments such as hypnosis, guided imagery, or meditation may help. Although these methods might not get rid of warts on their own, they can help with general health and maybe even speed up the healing process.

Methods for Treating Warts in Traditional Medicine

Common approaches for treating warts include applying salicylic acid-containing topical medicines or using freezing techniques, such as cryotherapy. When applied by trained medical personnel, these treatments are among the most popular and efficient methods for getting rid of warts.

Wart Patients' Use of Biofeedback and Relaxation Methods

Biofeedback is a method of teaching the mind to regulate physiological processes, such as heart rate and muscle tension. Biofeedback and relaxation techniques can assist patients in managing the pain and discomfort that often accompany wart removal treatments. However, these methods do not directly treat warts.

Pain Relief from Warts via Physical Therapy

Warts can be quite painful, especially on sensitive places like the feet or hands, but physical therapy procedures like massage and stretching exercises can help ease the pain and increase mobility.

The Use of Integrative Medicine in the Treatment of Warts

With an emphasis on a comprehensive approach to treatment, integrative medicine integrates traditional and alternative medical practices. To address the physical and mental components of wart management, a combination of established treatments like cryotherapy and complementary therapies like herbal medicines or acupuncture may be used for wart care.

For those looking for more comprehensive methods of wart treatment, each of these supplementary and alternative medicine options has its own set of advantages and things to think about. To guarantee a safe and effective therapy, it is vital to get advice from healthcare specialists and qualified practitioners when considering these choices.

CHAPTER 9

PROBLEMS WITH WARTS IN CERTAIN GROUPS

The Diagnosis and Treatment of Warts in Children

In children, warts manifest as a frequent skin condition. It is common practice for a healthcare provider to conduct a visual examination to make a diagnosis. The age, size, and location of the child's wart determine the treatment possibilities. Cryotherapy (freezing) and topical therapies like salicylic acid are frequently safe and helpful for youngsters. Surgery to remove a wart is an option for those with a particularly large or persistent wart, but it is typically reserved for extreme cases because of the pain it might induce.

Things to Think About and What to Do If You Have Warts While Pregnant

Several wart treatments should not be used during pregnancy because of the risks they pose to the developing baby. When trying to figure out what to do, it's important to talk to a doctor first. It is recommended to refrain from using topical therapies such as podophyllin and imiquimod when pregnant. Again, the dangers and benefits need to be carefully considered, but safer choices include cryotherapy and surgical removal under local anesthesia if necessary.

Warts in People With Reduced Immunity

Warts can be more common and difficult to treat in people with impaired immune systems, such as those living with HIV/AIDS or using immunosuppressive medication. Immunomodulatory therapy and topical meds are two examples of treatment techniques that aim to improve immune function. To detect problems early and intervene effectively, regular monitoring is crucial.

Management of Warts and Seniors

Factors including lowered immune function and slower healing make warts more difficult to control in the elderly. Possible treatments include topical medication and small surgical operations. Nevertheless, it is essential to carefully observe this population for any negative reactions and take into account the patient's general health condition.

Athletes and Active People and Warts

Because of the increased skin contact and perspiration accumulation, warts are common among athletes and active people. Wearing protective clothing and practicing excellent hygiene are prevention techniques that can be helpful. To treat the condition and keep it from coming back, a doctor may prescribe topical drugs and recommend changes to the patient's lifestyle.

LGBTQ+ Factors to Consider When Dealing with Genital Warts

No one is immune to genital warts, regardless of their sexual orientation or gender identity. Stigma, healthcare access, and conversations about sexual health are three areas where LGBTQ+ people may encounter unique obstacles. To meet their particular worries and requirements, it is vital to provide care that is culturally sensitive, use inclusive terminology, and create personalized treatment programs.

Warts and Their Treatment from a Cultural Perspective

Warts are regarded and treated differently depending on cultural beliefs and customs. Traditional treatments may be more acceptable in some cultures, or there may be social taboos around talking about skin problems. Providers of medical care owe it to their patients to be sensitive to their cultural backgrounds, and communicative, and to present them with treatment alternatives that take such factors into account.

Wart Treatment in Underdeveloped Nations

Developing nations may have restricted access to healthcare resources and treatment alternatives. Wart care in these contexts can be improved through community education, educating local healthcare providers, and the provision of cost-effective treatments, such as topical medicines. The availability of life-saving drugs and surgical procedures can be improved through partnerships with global organizations.

Warts' Effects on Mental Health in Different Groups

Mental health can be affected by warts, particularly if they are noticeable or last for a long time. People already at a disadvantage may feel this impact more acutely. A holistic approach to wart management that takes into account the needs of different populations includes mental health support, counseling, and the resolution of issues related to body image.

Customising Wart Treatments for Unique Instances

Age, immunological state, wart location, and patient preferences are some of the unique characteristics that need to be considered in each wart case to develop a personalized treatment. All of these factors should be considered by healthcare providers when they develop treatment programs. Successful outcomes for unique wart cases can be achieved through regular follow-ups, patient education, and treatment adaptation based on response and tolerance.

CHAPTER 10

RESEARCH AND TRENDS IN THE MANAGEMENT OF WARTS IN THE FUTURE

New Methods for Identifying Warts:

The human papillomavirus (HPV) is the most prevalent cause of warts, which are growths on the skin. Improvements in the efficiency and accuracy of diagnosing and treating warts have been made possible by advances in wart diagnostic procedures. Visual inspection and physical examination, two of the oldest forms of diagnosis, are still vital, although modern diagnostic tools frequently supplement them.

For example, dermoscopy enables for a detailed examination of skin lesions, which helps clinicians distinguish warts from other skin disorders. Atypical or complicated warts can be better diagnosed with the help of reflectance confocal microscopy (RCM), which offers real-time imaging of skin layers. If you believe that someone you know has HPV, you can confirm their diagnosis with a polymerase chain reaction (PCR) test.

Upcoming Innovative Therapies:

The emergence of new remedies is changing the face of wart therapy. While salicylic acid, cryotherapy, and surgical excision are still good alternatives, new ones are popping up to deal with problems including recurrence and patient pain.

Warts can be targeted and removed by the body's immune system through immunotherapy, which involves injecting antigens or immune response modifiers intralesionally. By utilizing a range of wavelengths, laser therapy can precisely target wart tissue while sparing the skin around it. The effectiveness of topical medicines that contain immune enhancers or antiviral chemicals in clearing warts is also being investigated.

Advancements in Wart Prevention Vaccination:

Vaccination as a means of preventing warts is an important topic of study. Several nations routinely immunise their citizens against certain kinds of human papillomavirus (HPV), including those that cause warts (HPV types 6 and 11). The effectiveness, longevity, and accessibility of vaccines are ongoing areas of focus.

Personalized Treatments for Different Kinds of Warts:

The best way to treat warts depends on the kind of warts you have. For instance, common warts on hands and plantar warts on feet may have distinct treatment responses. These differences are what motivated the development of targeted therapies, which provide tailored solutions for individual wart types.

Wart Research through the Use of Gene Therapy and Biotechnology:

The treatment of warts may soon be possible thanks to developments in biotechnology and gene therapy. Targeting and disrupting HPV genes within wart cells may be possible with gene editing techniques like CRISPR-Cas9, which could lead to long-lasting eradication. The efficacy and safety of wart therapies could be improved with the use of biotechnological advancements, such as new biomaterials and drug delivery systems.

A Revolution in Wart Management with AI:

Wart management methods are increasingly incorporating artificial intelligence (AI). By evaluating pictures and clinical data, AI algorithms can aid in the diagnosis of warts, making the diagnostic process more efficient and accurate. The use of machine learning algorithms to forecast response rates using patient data and historical results can also help with therapy selection.

Programs in Public Health to Eliminate Warts:

Wart eradication efforts rely heavily on public health activities. Prevention of warts, available treatments, and the significance of early intervention are all topics that education campaigns aim to bring to light. When people can afford medical care, they are more likely to seek prompt diagnosis and treatment, which in turn reduces the prevalence of warts in communities.

Wart Reduction Initiatives on a Global Scale:

The prevalence of warts is being addressed through international collaboration. Organizations on a global scale are actively working to standardize methods for diagnosing and treating warts, encourage cooperation among researchers, and fund immunization campaigns in neglected areas. To improve public health outcomes on a worldwide scale and reduce inequalities in the prevalence of warts, these initiatives are crucial.

Emphasizing the Patient's Needs in Wart Treatment:

Integrating patients into therapeutic decision-making and catering to their unique preferences and requirements are key tenets of patient-centered care. Treatment alternatives, side effects, and anticipated outcomes are all part of this strategy for wart management. Additionally, it stresses the need for continuous communication in tracking treatment outcomes, setting reasonable expectations, and guaranteeing patient happiness.

Future Hope for Wart Research and Development:

The treatment of warts is an area that needs further investigation in numerous important ways. Some of these areas that need attention include researching the function of the host immune system in wart clearance, creating more effective vaccines that cover more HPV strains, improving targeted therapy for particular wart types, and studying combination therapies to increase their effectiveness. Wart detection, treatment, and patient outcomes are anticipated to be even better with the integration of digital health solutions and the advancement of diagnostic technologies.